K.S. MERRILL

50+ At-Home Workouts

Get into great shape from the comfort of your own home

First edition

This book was professionally typeset on Reedsy.
Find out more at reedsy.com

Contents

1

Introduction

Exercising is an important part of life, no matter your age. Being physically active isn't only good for your physical health. While exercising will help keep your body strong and able to keep going for longer, it also has lasting effects on brain health, mental health, and emotional health. Everyone from your kids to your grandparents have something to gain from exercising! You don't need to go out and buy an expensive gym membership or get a personal trainer to effectively exercise. There are plenty of ways to exercise and stay in shape right in the comfort of your own home!

You should be exercising anywhere between 2 hours and 7 hours a week, depending on your personal goals. You don't need anything other than your own body weight to get a good workout at home but there are many exercises that are easy to do and great for you that involve some equipment. For the purpose of this book, necessary equipment includes a set of dumbbells that are an appropriate weight for you and resistance bands.

Getting Started

Before jumping into working out right away, it is important to stretch and to warm up. You'll want to stretch any muscle groups you plan on exercising and then do some cardio to get your heart rate up. Just as important as warming up is cooling down. A cool down allows your heart rate and your blood pressure to slowly return back to pre-exercise levels without crashing.

Warm-Ups & Cool Downs

Warming up will raise your heart rate and allow more blood flow to your extremities and muscle groups you will be exercising. Some warm ups may include:

- A light jog
- An easier version of the first set in your planned workout
- Some stretches
- Foam rolling
- Controlled Breathing
- Meditation

Stretching

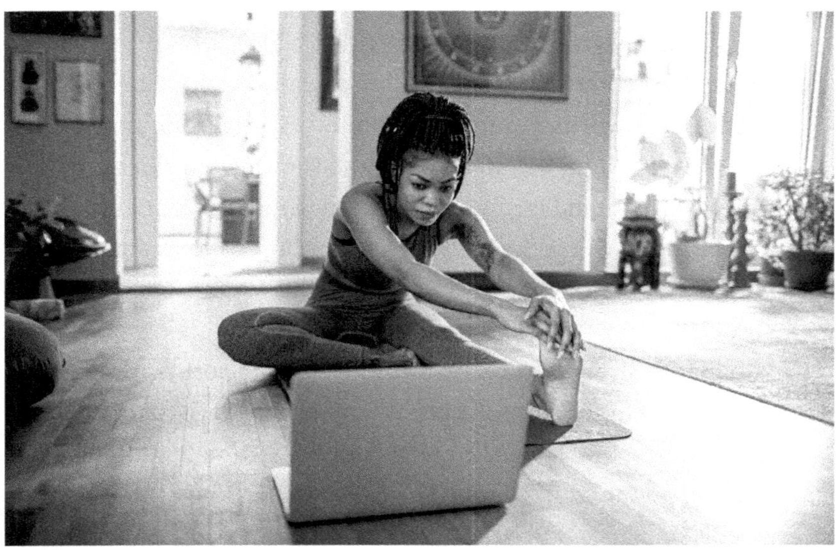

Stretching will help prevent injury and will help with soreness. It is very important to do before and after any exercise. Stretching is a crucial component of any fitness routine, as it helps improve flexibility, mobility, and overall range of motion. Stretching can also reduce muscle tension, improve circulation, and prevent injuries. There are several types of stretches, including static stretches and dynamic stretches. Here are some common stretches you can incorporate into your routine:

1. Hamstring Stretch (L-Stretch): Sit on the floor with one leg extended straight out in front of you and the other leg bent. Reach forward towards your toes, keeping your back straight, and hold

for 15-30 seconds. Repeat on the other leg.

2. Quadriceps Stretch: Stand tall and grab one foot behind you, pulling it towards your glutes while keeping your knees close together. Hold for 15-30 seconds and then switch sides.

3. Calf Stretch: Stand facing a wall with one foot in front of the other and both hands on the wall for support. Lean forward, keeping your back leg straight and your heel on the ground, until you feel a stretch in your calf. Hold for 15-30 seconds and then switch sides.

4. Hip Flexor Stretch: Kneel on one knee with the other foot in front of you, making sure your knee is bent at a 90-degree angle. Lean forward into the stretch, keeping your back straight, until you feel a stretch in the front of your hip. Hold for 15-30 seconds and then switch sides.

5. Chest Stretch: Stand tall with your arms extended straight out to the sides at shoulder height. Bring your arms behind you and clasp your hands together, gently squeezing your shoulder blades together. Hold for 15-30 seconds.

6. Triceps Stretch: Reach one arm overhead and bend it, bringing your hand down towards your upper back. Use your other hand to gently push your elbow towards your head until you feel a stretch in your triceps. Hold for 15-30 seconds and then switch sides.

7. Lower Back Stretch: Lie on your back with your knees bent and feet flat on the floor. Bring one knee towards your chest and hold it with both hands, gently pulling it towards you until you feel a stretch in your lower back. Hold for 15-30 seconds and then switch legs.

8. Shoulder Stretch: Stand tall and reach one arm across your body, using your other hand to gently press your arm towards you until you feel a stretch in your shoulder. Hold for 15-30 seconds and then switch sides.

Remember to stretch both sides of your body equally and to breathe deeply and slowly throughout each stretch. Stretching should never be painful, so if you feel any discomfort, ease off the stretch slightly. Incorporating stretching into your fitness routine can help improve your overall flexibility and mobility, leading to better performance and reduced risk of injury.

2

Arm Exercises

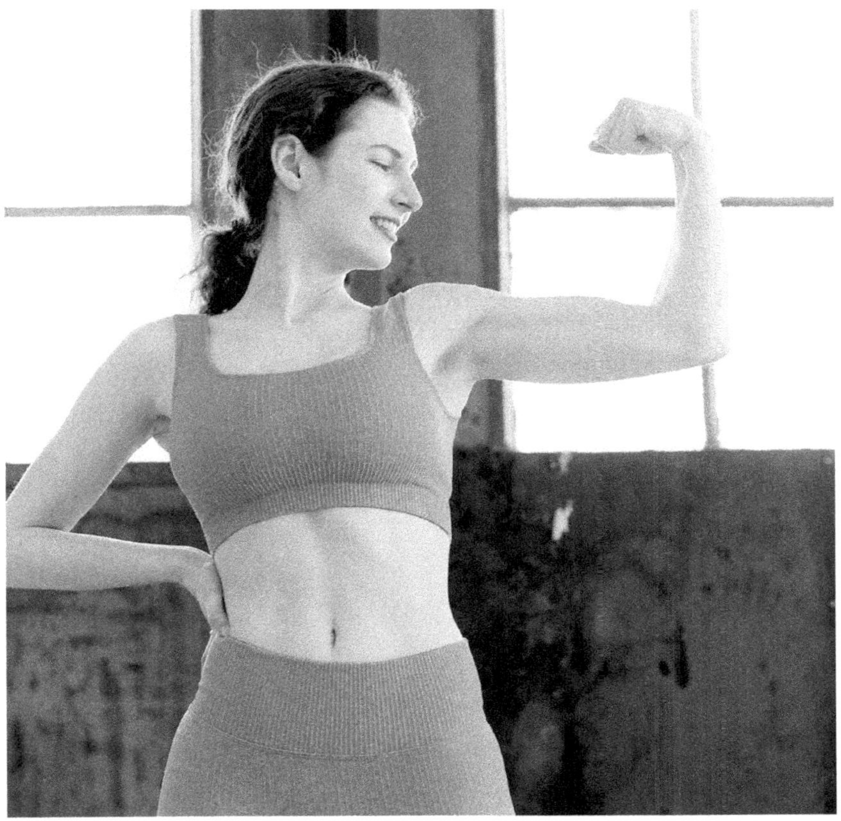

- Standard Push Ups

Standard push ups are a great body weight exercise. Start by laying down, supporting your body by your hands and toes. Keep your arms straight and hands shoulder width apart, legs extended and feet in-line with your hips. Lower your body until your chest almost touches the floor then push yourself back up to return to the starting position. That is one push up. Standard push ups target your arms, shoulders, and chest.

• Wide Set Push Ups

Wide set push ups are a variation of the standard push up. You begin with your hands placed wider than shoulder width apart. Again, you will lower your body until your chest almost touches the floor then push yourself back up to return to the starting position. Wide set push ups target the arm, shoulder, and chest muscles with an added emphasis on the outer chest muscles.

• Balance Push ups

Balance push ups are also known as stability ball push ups or swiss ball push ups. In this variation you place your hands on a ball such as a soccer ball or basketball. As you lower your body, focus on keeping the ball still and in the same spot without wobbling. This exercise targets your arm, shoulder, chest and core muscles with an added emphasis on the core.

• Tricep Dips

Tricep dips focus on your triceps, the muscle group on the back of your upper arm behind your biceps. Start by sitting on a chair or bench, grip the front of the seat with your hands and move forward so your back is in front of your hands. Make sure your knees are bent at 90 degrees. Lower your body by bending your elbows until your upper arms are parallel to the floor then raise your body back up, straightening your arms. During this exercise, only use your legs to balance yourself, don't use your legs to help push back up. Tricep dips will effectively strengthen and help define your tricep muscles.

- Pull Ups

Pull ups are a great upper body workout but can also be challenging. Pull ups are performed by grabbing onto a horizontal bar above your head with an outward grip (palms facing away from you) and pulling your body weight up until your chin clears the bar. Then return to the starting position in a controlled way. Try to avoid swinging or kicking your legs to get the most out of this exercise. Pull ups mainly target your upper back muscle groups but also engage your biceps, shoulders, and forearms. To make this exercise a bit easier, you can use resistance bands wrapped around the bar and under your feet. The resistance band will help pull you up because of the elasticity, but be careful not to let it slip off of your feet.

- Bicep Curls

Bicep curls are a weighted exercise that isolates your biceps, the muscle on the front of your upper arm. Grab dumbbells of an appropriate weight in each hand and start with your arms fully extended down by your sides with an outward facing grip. Starting with one arm, bring the dumbbell up towards your shoulders by bending your elbow trying not to swing your body or use your shoulder muscles at all. Once at the top of the curl, pause briefly before lowering the weight back down slowly and controlled. There are many variations to the bicep curl to isolate the bicep muscle such as a "Hammer Curl" where you hold the dumbbells with an inward facing grip. As you curl the dumbbell, it will resemble the swing of a hammer.

- Tricep Kickbacks

Tricep kickbacks are a weighted exercise that isolates your triceps. Start by grabbing an appropriate weight of dumbbells in each hand. Begin by standing with your feet shoulder-width apart. Bend your knees and slightly hinge forward at your waist bringing your torso as close to parallel with the floor as possible. Hold the dumbbells with your palms facing inward and keep your elbows close to your side to maximize tricep engagement. Bend your arms so your upper arms are parallel to the floor and your elbow is at 90 degrees. Push the dumbbell back, extending your arm, until your arm is straight behind you and parallel with the floor. Hold the weight there briefly before bringing the weight back slowly and controlled, bending your elbow at 90 degrees.

- Overhead Tricep Extensions

Overhead tricep extensions target your triceps' long head using a single Dumbbell or an EZ Bar. Sit on a chair or a bench with your back straight and upright. Hold the weight of your choosing above your head with your arms extended. Slowly lower the weight behind your head keeping your elbows by your head bending them until your forearms are parallel to the floor or until you feel your triceps stretching. Bring the weight back following the same path in which you lowered the weight fully extending your arms and contracting your triceps at the top.

- Lateral Raise

Lateral raises, also called shoulder flys, are an exercise that targets the lateral deltoids which are the diamond shaped muscles on sides of the shoulders. Start by standing with your feet shoulder-width apart, holding a dumbbell of appropriate weight in each hand. Keeping your arms straight (but not locked) with a slight bend at the elbows, lift the dumbbells out to the sides until your arms are parallel to the floor. Your arms should be in line with your shoulders forming a "T" shape with your body. Try to keep your body still and focus on lifting the weight with your shoulders and not a swinging motion. Hold the dumbbells at the top for a brief moment before lowering your arms back down to your sides slowly and controlled.

3

Chest Exercises

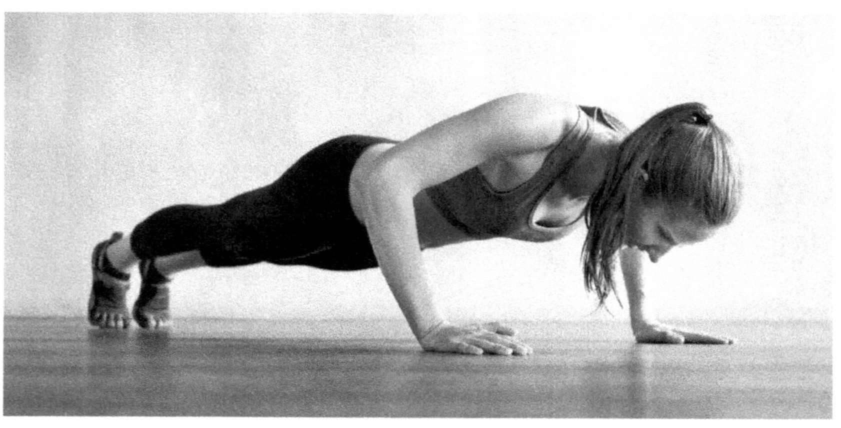

• One-Leg Push Ups

One-leg push ups are also called single-leg push ups or unilateral push ups. Start by beginning in the standard push up position, hands shoulder-width apart and your body in a straight line from head to heels. Lift one leg a few inches off the ground and hold it there. This exercise will engage the core and glutes more than a classic push up. Lower your body until your chest almost touches the floor keeping your elbows close to your side. Push your body back up, fully extending your arms. Make sure you switch which leg is in the air and which leg is on the ground each set, do an even amount of sets.

- Diamond Push Ups

Diamond push ups are also called triangle push ups or close grip push ups. Start by beginning in the standard push up position, but bring your hands in directly below your chest forming a triangle with your index fingers and thumbs. Keep your feet shoulder-width apart and your body in a straight line from head to heel. Lower your body with your elbows bending out to your sides until your chest almost touches your hands. Push your body back up, pressing through your palms and fully extending your elbows. Diamond push ups target your chest, triceps, and shoulders to a greater extent.

- Incline Push Ups

Incline push ups begin with finding a stable platform elevated from the ground such as a bench, step, or chair. Place your hands on the elevated platform shoulder-width apart and extend your legs out behind you keeping your body in a straight line from head to heels. Lower your body until your chest almost touches the elevated platform, bending at the elbows keeping your elbows close to your sides and your body straight. Push back up through your palms until your arms are fully extended. Incline push ups are less challenging than a standard push up but they focus on the lower chest muscles.

- Decline Push Ups

Decline push ups begin with finding a stable elevated platform such as a bench, step, or chair. Place your feet on the elevated platform shoulder-width apart when in standard push up position. Place your hands on the floor shoulder-width apart. Your body should be parallel to the ground or your head should be closer to the ground than your feet. Lower your body keeping your elbows close to your sides until your chest or your head almost touch the floor, then push back up through your palms until your arms are fully extended. Decline push ups target the upper chest muscles more directly.

- Offset Push Ups

Offset push ups, also called staggered push ups, isolate one arm and one side of your chest, making it work harder than the other side. Begin by finding a stable surface that is no taller than the length of your forearm. You can use a yoga block, step, or stool. You can even use a stack of books or something similar. Place one hand on the elevated surface and the other on the floor shoulder-width apart. Place your feet on the floor extended behind you also shoulder-width apart. Lower your body keeping your elbows by your sides and your body in a straight line until your elevated hand almost touches your shoulder. Push back up through your palms until the arm on the floor is fully extended. Offset push ups help improve balance and stability by challenging your chest, shoulder, and tricep muscles asymmetrically.

- Dumbbell Chest Press

Dumbbell chest press, also called chest press or dumbbell press, targets the chest, shoulder, tricep muscles. Lie down on a flat bench with a dumbbell of appropriate weight in each hand. Keep your feet planted firmly on the ground in front of you and keep your back flat against the bench. Hold the dumbbells above your chest with your arms fully extended and your palms facing outward. Lower the dumbbells towards your chest, bending at your elbows. Press the dumbbells back up to the starting position. Keep your wrists straight and avoid locking your elbows when fully extended. Focus on maintaining a slow and controlled movement throughout the exercise. Avoid any jerking or swinging motions to avoid injuries.

You can perform the dumbbell chest press on an incline bench to target the upper chest muscles or on a decline bench to target the lower chest muscles.

- Chest Fly

The chest fly is also known as a dumbbell fly. The chest fly is an isolation exercise that primarily targets the chest muscles. It also engages the shoulders and the triceps to a lesser extent. Lie down on a flat bench with a dumbbell of appropriate weight in each hand. Keep your feet planted firmly on the ground in front of you and keep your back flat against the bench. With a slight bend in your elbows, slowly lower your arms in a wide arc until your arms are parallel to the floor or slightly below. Keep your elbows in line with your shoulders during the movement. Press the dumbbells back up to the starting position. Exhale as you lift the weights focusing on contracting the chest muscles. Keep your wrists straight and avoid locking your elbows when returned to the starting position. Focus on maintaining a slow and controlled movement throughout the exercise. Avoid any jerking or swinging motions to avoid injuries.

You can perform the chest fly on an incline bench to target the upper chest muscles or on a decline bench to target the lower chest muscles.

4

Core and Abdominal Exercises

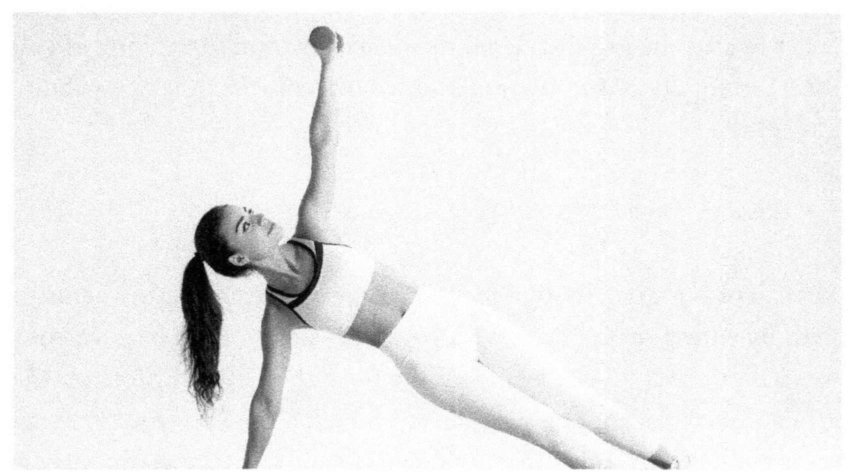

- Plank

The plank is a great exercise for building core strength, stability, and endurance. The plank is a fundamental body weight exercise that targets the abdominal, and lower back muscles. Start by getting into a push up position, hands and feet shoulder-width apart and your body in a straight line from head to heels. You can choose to perform the plank on your forearms or on your hands. Being on your forearms is more challenging and on your hands is less challenging. If you choose to be on your forearms make sure your elbows are directly beneath your shoulders. Engage your core by trying to bring your rib cage to your hips while keeping your body straight. Squeezing your glutes will help you maintain proper form. Avoid swaying or bouncing, keep your neck straight in line with your spine and keep your face towards the ground. Hold the plank position for as long as you can. Aim for 20-30 seconds at first then increase the time as you build strength.

- Russian Twists

Russian twists target the obliques which are on the side of the abdomen. Start by sitting on the floor with your knees bent. Lean back so your torso is at about 45 degrees from the floor then lift your feet off the ground so you balance on your lower back. You can keep your heels on the ground if you need more balance and stability, but if you can balance without your feet it is better. Engage your core to balance and stabilize yourself in order to maintain correct posture and proper alignment. Hold a dumbbell, medicine ball, or weighted plate with both hands in between your chest and your knees. Bring the weight down to your right side so it almost touches the floor next to your hip. Twist at your waist and keep your back as straight as you can. Then from the right side, pass through the center starting position and bring the weight down to your left so it almost touches the floor next to your hip. Bring the weight back to the starting position, that is one russian twist. Focus on maintaining a constant speed throughout the repetition without stopping or jerking or swinging. Maintain control over the weight you're using and don't twist too fast. Russian twists will strengthen your core and help balance and stability.

- Bicycle Kicks

Bicycle kicks, also known as bicycle crunches or bicycles, target the abdomen, obliques, and hip flexors. Lay flat on your back with your legs extended and your hands gently supporting your head. Lift your legs off the ground and bend them to 90 degrees. Start by extending your right leg out and bringing your left knee towards your chest. Twist your torso bringing your right elbow to your left knee. Reverse the motion straightening your left leg while bringing your right knee towards your chest. Twist your torso the other way bringing your left elbow to your right knee. Maintain a slow controlled movement throughout the exercise and keep your core engaged to avoid any rocking or shifting. Bicycle kicks are a great exercise to help improve core strength and stability.

- Mountain Climbers

Mountain climbers are a great exercise that targets the core, shoulders, and hip flexors. They also engage the chest, arms and legs. Start in the plank position with your hands directly below your shoulders and your body in a straight line from head to heels. Begin by bringing your right knee up into your chest, keep your toes pointed and your foot off the ground. As you return your foot to the starting position, simultaneously bring your left foot up into your chest keeping your toes pointed and your foot off the ground. Continue alternating legs in a rhythmic, running motion. Keep your hips low and your spine in line, aim for a steady and fluid motion. Avoid any jerking or bouncing.

- Butterfly Kicks

Butterfly kicks are a core exercise that targets the lower abdominal muscles, hip flexors, and inner thighs. Lie on your back with your arms by your sides. Keep your legs straight and together. Lift your legs off the ground a few inches while keeping them straight. Begin by moving your right leg up and your left leg down in an alternating fluttering motion. Keep your legs straight as you alternate kicking up and down. Focus on maintaining a controlled and steady motion throughout the exercise. Avoid any jerky or swinging movements, and keep your core engaged to prevent your lower back from lifting off the ground. You can place your hands under your lower back to help keep your tailbone off the ground, or you can get a mat to help cushion your body. It's also a bit easier with your hands under your lower back as support if it is too challenging otherwise. Adjust the pace and intensity of the butterfly kicks to match your fitness level and goals. You can increase the speed for a more intense workout or slow it down to focus on controlled movements and muscle engagement. Perform butterfly kicks for a set duration, such as 30 seconds to 1 minute.

Butterfly kicks are an effective exercise for targeting the lower abdominal muscles and hip flexors while also engaging the inner thighs. They can help improve core strength, stability, and endurance when performed regularly and with proper form.

- Leg Lifts

Leg lifts, also known as leg raises, are a classic abdominal exercise that primarily targets the lower abdominal muscles. Lie flat on your back on a mat with your arms by your sides and your palms facing down. Keep your legs straight and together. Keeping your legs straight, lift them off the ground until they are perpendicular to the floor or as high as you can comfortably lift them. Your feet should be flexed, and your toes pointing towards the ceiling. Slowly lower your legs back down towards the ground, maintaining control and keeping your lower back pressed into the ground. Avoid letting your feet touch the ground between repetitions to keep tension on the abdominal muscles. Focus on lifting your legs using your lower abdominal muscles rather than swinging them up with momentum. Only lift your legs as high as you can while maintaining control and without arching your lower back off the ground. Perform leg lifts at a controlled pace, focusing on proper form and muscle engagement. You can adjust the intensity by slowing down the movement or adding ankle weights for added resistance. Leg lifts are an effective exercise for targeting the lower abdominal muscles and improving core strength and stability.

- Toe Taps

Toe taps are an explosive abdominal exercise. Start by lying flat on a mat with your arms extending up past your head, palms facing upwards, and your legs together extending down. Keeping your legs together, lift them a few inches off the ground. Your feet should be flexed, and your toes pointing toward the ceiling. In a single movement, lift your legs up until they are perpendicular to the floor or as high as you can comfortably lift them. Bring your hands up from above your head in a wide arc, keeping your arms straight, and tap your toes in the air above you. Lower your arms and legs back down and keep your heels a few inches off the ground. Focus on lifting your legs with your lower abdominal muscles rather than swinging them up with momentum. Focus on engaging your core when lifting your arms to your toes. Toe taps are an effective exercise for strengthening your core and hip flexors.

- One-arm Plank

The one-arm plank or side-plank, primarily targets the oblique muscles, which are located on the sides of the abdomen, as well as the shoulders, hips, and core stabilizing muscles. Start by lying on your side with your legs extended and stacked on top of each other. Place your elbow directly beneath your shoulder on the side that is facing upward. Your forearm should be perpendicular to your body, and your hand should be flat on the ground. Extend your legs fully, and engage your core muscles to lift your body off the ground. Lift your hips off the ground, creating a straight line from your head to your heels. Your body should form a diagonal plank position, with your weight supported by your forearm and the side of your bottom foot. Focus on balancing your body and maintaining stability throughout the exercise. Keep your hips lifted and avoid letting them sag towards the ground. Hold the one-arm plank position for a set duration, such as 20-30 seconds to start, or for as long as you can maintain proper form. Keep your breathing steady and focus on engaging your core muscles throughout the hold. After completing the desired duration on one side, lower your hips back down to the ground and switch to the other side to perform the one-arm plank on the opposite side. The one-arm plank is an effective exercise for strengthening the oblique muscles and improving overall core stability. Focus on maintaining proper form and alignment throughout the movement to maximize the benefits and minimize the risk of injury.

- Inchworm

The inchworm exercise is a dynamic full-body movement that targets the core, shoulders, arms, hamstrings, and hip flexors. Stand by standing tall with your feet hip-width apart and your arms by your sides. Bend forward at your hips and lower your torso towards the ground, reaching your hands towards the floor. Keep your legs straight or slightly bent if needed to maintain comfort. Once your hands reach the ground, walk them forward away from your body, keeping your legs as straight as possible. Continue walking your hands out until you are in a plank position, with your body forming a straight line from head to heels. Hold the plank position for a brief moment, engaging your core muscles to maintain stability and alignment. From the plank position, slowly walk your hands back towards your feet, keeping your legs as straight as possible. As you walk your hands back, focus on keeping your core engaged and maintaining a flat back. Repeat the sequence, walking out to plank and walking back to the starting position. Focus on maintaining a smooth and controlled movement throughout the exercise, avoiding any jerky or rushed motions. Keep your core engaged and your back flat during the plank position to maximize the benefits and protect your lower back. If you have tight hamstrings, you can bend your knees slightly during the forward fold to make the movement more comfortable. As you become more comfortable with the exercise, you can increase the intensity by walking your hands out further or adding a push up when in the plank position. The inchworm exercise is a versatile movement that can be incorporated into your warm-up routine, used as part of a dynamic stretching sequence, or included in a full-body workout for added core and upper body strengthening.

- Shoulder Taps

Shoulder taps are a dynamic core exercise that also engage the shoulders, arms, and chest. Begin in a plank position with your hands directly beneath your shoulders and your body forming a straight line from head to heels. Your feet should be hip-width apart to provide a stable base. Lift your right hand off the ground and tap your left shoulder with your right hand. Return your right hand to the starting position, then lift your left hand off the ground and tap your right shoulder with your left hand. Alternate tapping each shoulder while maintaining a stable plank position. Focus on maintaining a stable plank position throughout the exercise, avoiding any twisting or rocking of the hips. Keep your core engaged and your body in a straight line from head to heels. Perform shoulder taps at a controlled pace, focusing on proper form and muscle engagement. You can adjust the intensity by increasing the speed of the taps or slowing down to focus on stability. You could also tap your knee after tapping the corresponding shoulders. Shoulder taps are an effective exercise for improving core stability, shoulder strength, and coordination. They can be incorporated into your workout routine as part of a core circuit or performed as a standalone exercise. Focus on maintaining proper form and control throughout the movement to maximize the benefits and minimize the risk of injury.

5

Back Exercises

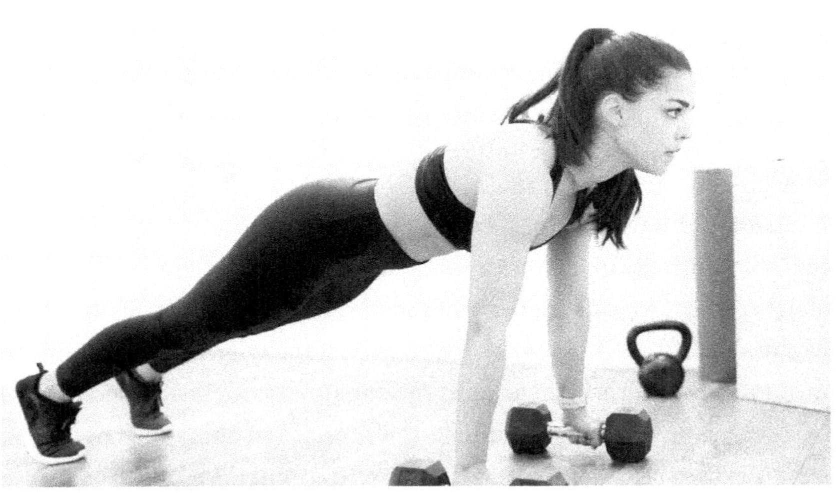

- Resistance Band Pull-apart

The resistance band pull-apart is an excellent exercise for targeting the muscles of the upper back, specifically the rear deltoids, rhomboids, and traps. It's also effective for improving shoulder stability and posture. Stand with your feet hip-width apart and hold a resistance band with both hands in front of you. Choose a resistance band with an appropriate level of tension for your strength level. Hold the resistance band with an overhand grip, keeping your hands slightly wider than shoulder-width apart. Ensure that there is tension on the band when your arms are extended in front of you. Extend your arms straight out in front of you at shoulder height, with your elbows slightly bent. Keep your chest up, shoulders back, and core engaged throughout the exercise. Pull the resistance band apart by squeezing your shoulder blades together and driving your elbows out to the sides. Focus on engaging the muscles of your upper back and keeping your arms straight throughout the movement. At the end of the movement, your hands should be at shoulder height, and the resistance band should be stretched across your chest. Pause for a moment to feel the contraction in your upper back muscles. Slowly return to the starting position by bringing your hands back together in front of you. Maintain control and tension in the resistance band throughout the movement. The resistance band pull-apart can be performed as part of a warm-up routine to activate the muscles of the upper back and shoulders, or as a standalone exercise to strengthen and tone these muscles. It's important to use proper form and technique to maximize effectiveness and prevent injury. Adjust the tension of the resistance band by choosing a band with more or less resistance, or by adjusting your grip width.

- Back Extensions

The lying down back extension, also known as the prone back extension, is an exercise that targets the muscles of the lower back, hamstrings, and glutes. Start by lying face down on a mat or flat surface with your legs straight and your arms extended overhead, palms facing down. Your body should be fully extended. Lift your upper body off the ground by contracting your lower back muscles. Keep your neck in a neutral position and avoid straining your neck by looking too far forward. As you lift your upper body, also squeeze your glutes to help support your lower back and maintain stability. At the top of the movement, your body should form a straight line from your head to your heels, with your hips pressed into the ground. Pause for a moment to squeeze your lower back muscles. Lower your upper body back down to the starting position in a controlled manner. Perform the desired number of repetitions, aiming for 10-15 reps, depending on your fitness level and goals. The lying down back extension is a low-impact exercise that can help improve lower back strength, flexibility, and endurance. It's important to use controlled movements and avoid hyperextending your lower back at the top of the movement.

• Quadruped Single-arm Dumbbell Row

The quadruped single-arm dumbbell row is a compound exercise that primarily targets the muscles of the back, including the latissimus dorsi, rhomboids, and rear deltoids, while also engaging the core and stabilizing muscles. Start in a quadruped position (on your hands and knees) on a mat or bench, with your hands directly beneath your shoulders and your knees directly beneath your hips. Hold a dumbbell in one hand, with your palm facing your body, and let your arm hang straight down towards the floor. Engage your core muscles. This will help stabilize your torso throughout the exercise and prevent excessive twisting or arching of the lower back. Keeping your core engaged and your back flat, pull the dumbbell up towards your rib cage, bending your elbow and retracting your shoulder blade. Keep your elbow close to your body and your wrist straight throughout the movement. At the top of the movement, squeeze your back muscles and hold for a moment to maximize muscle activation. Slowly lower the dumbbell back down towards the floor, extending your arm fully but maintaining tension in your back muscles. Perform the desired number of repetitions on one side before switching to the other side. Aim for 8-12 repetitions per arm, depending on your fitness level and goals. Throughout the exercise, focus on maintaining stability in your core and avoiding any rotation or shifting of your hips. Keep your shoulders square and your spine in a neutral position. The quadruped single-arm dumbbell row is an effective exercise for building strength and muscle mass in the back while also improving core stability and balance. It can be incorporated into your back workout routine or used as a unilateral exercise to address muscle imbalances between the left and right sides of the body. Adjust the weight of the dumbbell to suit your strength level and ensure proper form throughout the exercise.

- Single-arm Dumbbell Row

The single-arm dumbbell row is a classic strength training exercise that primarily targets the muscles of the upper back, including the latissimus dorsi, rhomboids, and rear deltoids, as well as the biceps and forearms. Begin by standing with your feet shoulder-width apart, holding a dumbbell in one hand. You can also perform this exercise with your knee and hand supported on a bench or other elevated surface, which is called a supported dumbbell row. For the standing version, hinge at your hips to bend forward, keeping your back straight and your chest up. Engage your core muscles. This will help stabilize your torso throughout the exercise and prevent excessive arching of your lower back. With the dumbbell hanging straight down towards the floor, pull the dumbbell up towards your rib cage, bending your elbow and retracting your shoulder blade. Keep your elbow close to your body and your wrist straight throughout the movement. At the top of the movement, squeeze your back muscles and hold for a moment to maximize muscle activation. Slowly lower the dumbbell back down towards the floor, extending your arm fully but maintaining tension in your back muscles. Perform the desired number of repetitions on one side before switching to the other side. Aim for 8-12 repetitions per arm, depending on your fitness level and goals. Throughout the exercise, focus on maintaining stability in your core and avoiding any rotation or shifting of your hips. Keep your shoulders square and your spine in a neutral position. The single-arm dumbbell row is an effective exercise for building strength and muscle mass in the upper back while also improving grip strength and stability. It can be incorporated into your back workout routine or used as a unilateral exercise to address muscle imbalances between the left and right sides of the body. Adjust the weight of the dumbbell to suit your strength level and ensure proper form throughout the exercise.

- Bent Row

The bent-over row is a compound exercise that primarily targets the muscles of the upper back, including the latissimus dorsi, rhomboids, and rear deltoids, as well as the biceps and forearms. Stand with your feet hip-width apart, holding a barbell or dumbbells with an overhand grip (palms facing towards you) at about shoulder-width apart. You can also use an underhand grip if preferred. Bend your knees slightly and hinge at your hips to lean forward, keeping your back straight and your chest up. Your torso should be at about a 45-degree angle to the floor. Engage your core muscles. This will help stabilize your torso throughout the exercise and prevent excessive arching of your lower back. With the weights hanging straight down towards the floor, pull the weights up towards your rib cage, bending your elbows and retracting your shoulder blades. Keep your elbows close to your body and your wrists straight throughout the movement. At the top of the movement, squeeze your back muscles and hold for a moment to maximize muscle activation. Slowly lower the weights back down towards the floor, extending your arms fully but maintaining tension in your back muscles. Perform the desired number of repetitions, aiming for 8-12 reps, depending on your fitness level and goals. Throughout the exercise, focus on maintaining stability in your core and avoiding any rotation or shifting of your hips. Keep your shoulders square and your spine in a neutral position. The bent-over row is an effective exercise for building strength and muscle mass in the upper back, as well as improving posture and stability. It can be incorporated into your back workout routine or used as a compound movement to target multiple muscle groups simultaneously. Adjust the weight of the barbell or dumbbells to suit your strength level and ensure proper form throughout the exercise.

- Renegade Dumbbell Row

The renegade dumbbell row is a challenging exercise that targets the muscles of the upper back, shoulders, and core. Start in a plank position with your hands holding a pair of dumbbells, palms facing each other, and your hands directly beneath your shoulders. Your feet should be hip-width apart to provide stability. Engage your core muscles to keep your body in a straight line from head to heels. With the dumbbells in hand, perform a rowing motion with one arm, pulling the dumbbell up towards your rib cage while keeping your elbow close to your body. Focus on squeezing your shoulder blade towards your spine to engage the muscles of your upper back. As you row with one arm, keep your hips and shoulders square to the ground to prevent rotation of your torso. Engage your core muscles to maintain stability and prevent your hips from rocking side to side. Slowly lower the dumbbell back down towards the floor, extending your arm fully but maintaining tension in your back muscles. After completing a row with one arm, lower the dumbbell back to the floor and repeat the rowing motion with the opposite arm. Continue alternating arms for the desired number of repetitions, aiming for 8-12 reps per arm. The renegade dumbbell row is an advanced exercise that challenges both upper body strength and core stability. It targets the muscles of the back, shoulders, and core. Start with lighter weights and gradually increase the resistance as you become stronger and more proficient with the movement.

- Reverse Fly

The reverse fly is an isolation exercise that targets the muscles of the upper back, particularly the rear deltoids (posterior deltoids), as well as the rhomboids and traps. Begin by standing with your feet shoulder-width apart, holding a dumbbell in each hand. Bend your knees slightly and hinge forward at your hips, keeping your back straight and your chest up. Your torso should be at about a 45-degree angle to the floor. Engage your core muscles to help stabilize your torso throughout the exercise and prevent excessive arching of your lower back. With your palms facing each other, extend your arms straight down towards the floor, allowing the dumbbells to hang directly beneath your shoulders. Raise both arms out to the sides in a wide arc, leading with your elbows and squeezing your shoulder blades together at the top of the movement. Keep a slight bend in your elbows throughout the exercise to reduce stress on the joints. At the top of the movement, pause for a moment to squeeze your shoulder blades together and maximize muscle activation in the upper back. Slowly lower the dumbbells back down towards the starting position, maintaining control and tension in your upper back muscles. Throughout the exercise, focus on maintaining stability in your core and avoiding any swinging motions or using momentum. Keep your shoulders square and your spine in a neutral position. The reverse fly is an effective exercise for targeting the muscles of the upper back and improving posture. It can be incorporated into your back workout routine or used as a supplementary exercise to target the rear deltoids and balance out the muscles of the shoulder girdle. Adjust the weight of the dumbbells to suit your strength level and ensure proper form throughout the exercise.

6

Glute Exercises

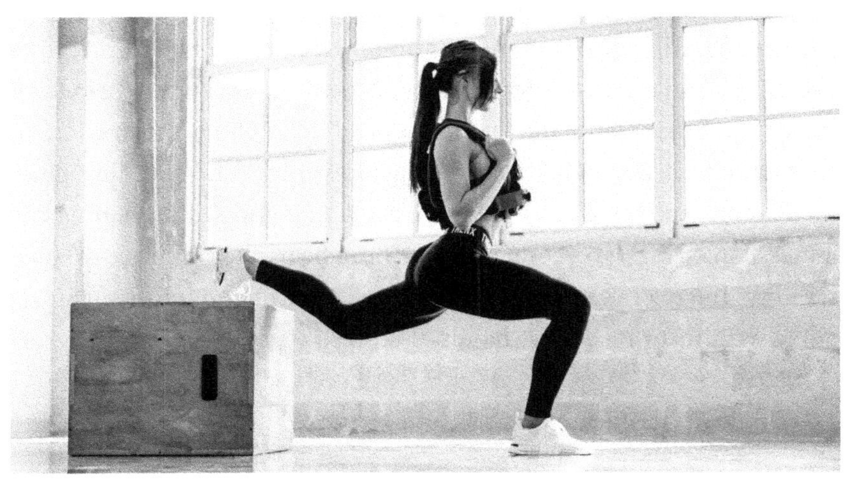

- Standing Glute Kickback

The standing glute kickback is a great exercise to target the gluteus maximus, hamstrings, and core muscles. Stand tall with your feet hip-width apart. Engage your core muscles to maintain stability throughout the exercise. Shift your weight onto one leg while slightly bending the knee of the supporting leg. This will be your starting position. Keeping your back straight, hinge forward at your hips while simultaneously extending your other leg straight back behind you. Focus on squeezing your glutes at the top of the movement to fully engage the muscles. Avoid arching your back or swinging your leg. Keep the movement controlled and deliberate to maximize muscle activation. Slowly lower your extended leg back down to the starting position, maintaining control throughout the movement. Perform the desired number of repetitions on one leg before switching to the other leg. Aim for 10-15 reps per leg, depending on your fitness level. Keep your hips square and facing forward throughout the movement to ensure that both glutes are engaged evenly. The standing glute kickback is an effective exercise for targeting and strengthening the glutes, hamstrings, and core muscles. It can be used to improve balance, stability, and overall lower body strength. Adjust the intensity by using ankle weights or resistance bands, if desired.

- Donkey Kickback

Donkey kickbacks, also known as donkey kicks, are an effective exercise for targeting the glutes and hamstrings. Start on your hands and knees on a mat or floor. Position your hands directly beneath your shoulders and your knees directly beneath your hips. Keep your back flat and your core engaged throughout the exercise. Engage your core to help stabilize your torso and prevent excessive arching of your lower back. Keeping your knee bent at a 90-degree angle, exhale as you lift one leg up towards the ceiling, pressing your heel towards the sky. Focus on squeezing your glutes at the top of the movement to fully engage the muscles. At the top of the movement, pause for a moment to squeeze your glutes before lowering your leg back down to the starting position. Perform the desired number of repetitions on one leg before switching to the other leg. Aim for 10-15 reps per leg, depending on your fitness level. Keep your hips square and facing down towards the ground throughout the movement to ensure that both glutes are engaged evenly. Keep the movement controlled and deliberate to maximize muscle activation and prevent swinging or momentum. Donkey kickbacks are a great exercise for targeting the glutes and hamstrings, and they can be easily incorporated into your lower body workout routine. Adjust the intensity by adding ankle weights or resistance bands, if desired.

- "Good morning"

Good mornings are a compound exercise primarily targeting the muscles of the lower back, hamstrings, and glutes. Begin by standing with your feet shoulder-width apart, holding a pair of dumbbells at shoulder height. You can also perform this exercise with a barbell or a resistance band for added resistance. Engage your core muscles to help stabilize your torso throughout the exercise and prevent excessive arching of your lower back. Keeping your back straight and your chest up, hinge forward at your hips while simultaneously bending your knees slightly. Lower your torso towards the ground, allowing it to come forward until it is roughly parallel to the floor. Your back should remain flat throughout the movement. Push your hips back and return to the starting position by squeezing your glutes and hamstrings. Focus on driving your hips forward to bring your torso back to an upright position. Throughout the exercise, focus on maintaining stability in your core and avoiding any rounding or excessive arching of your lower back. Good mornings are an effective exercise for strengthening the muscles of the lower back, hamstrings, and glutes, as well as improving hip mobility and overall posterior chain strength. Make sure to use proper form and start with lighter weights before progressing to heavier loads to minimize the risk of injury.

- Banded Glute Bridge

Banded glute bridges are a variation of the traditional glute bridge exercise that adds resistance using a resistance band to further target and strengthen the glutes. Begin by lying on your back on a mat with your knees bent and your feet flat on the ground. Place a resistance band just above your knees and pull it taut so that there is resistance when you push against it. Engage your core muscles to help stabilize your torso throughout the exercise and protect your lower back. Press through your heels and lift your hips towards the ceiling, squeezing your glutes at the top of the movement. Keep your knees aligned with your hips and your feet flat on the ground. Throughout the movement, actively push against the resistance band with your knees to engage the gluteus medius and maximus muscles even more. At the top of the movement, your body should form a straight line from your shoulders to your knees. Hold the top position for a moment to maximize muscle activation. Slowly lower your hips back down towards the ground, maintaining tension in the glutes and keeping the resistance band engaged. Banded glute bridges are an effective exercise for strengthening the glutes, hamstrings, and core muscles, as well as improving hip stability and mobility. Incorporate them into your lower body workout routine to add variety and challenge to your training. Adjust the resistance of the band as needed to suit your strength level and goals.

- Curtsy Lunge

The curtsy lunge is a variation of the traditional lunge exercise that targets the muscles of the lower body, including the quadriceps, glutes, hamstrings, and adductors. Begin by standing tall with your feet hip-width apart and your hands on your hips or by your sides. Take a big step diagonally backward with your right foot, crossing it behind your left leg. Aim to place your right foot slightly outside of your left foot. Lower your body down towards the ground by bending both knees, keeping your chest up and your back straight. Your left knee should be aligned with your left ankle, and your right knee should point towards the ground. Lower your body until your right knee almost touches the ground, or as far down as is comfortable for you. Keep your weight evenly distributed between both legs. Push through your left heel to return to the starting position, driving your right foot back to its starting position. Repeat the movement on the opposite side, stepping diagonally backward with your left foot and crossing it behind your right leg. Continue alternating sides for the desired number of repetitions, aiming for 8-12 reps per leg. The curtsy lunge is a great exercise for targeting the muscles of the lower body, particularly the glutes and outer thighs. It also challenges balance and stability, making it an effective functional exercise. You can perform curtsy lunges to strengthen and tone your legs. Adjust the depth and intensity of the movement by modifying the size of your step and the weight used.

- Fire Hydrant

The fire hydrant exercise, also known as hip abduction, is a great way to target the muscles of the outer thighs (abductors) and glutes. Begin on your hands and knees on a mat or the floor. Your hands should be directly under your shoulders and your knees directly under your hips. Keep your spine neutral and your core engaged throughout the exercise. Tighten your abdominal muscles to help stabilize your torso and prevent your lower back from arching. Keeping your knee bent at a 90-degree angle, exhale as you lift one knee out to the side, away from your body, while keeping your hips and shoulders square to the ground. Imagine you're a dog at a fire hydrant, lifting your leg to urinate. Avoid arching your back or leaning to one side as you lift your leg. Keep the movement controlled and deliberate, focusing on using the muscles of the outer thigh and glute to lift your leg. At the top of the movement, pause for a moment and squeeze your glutes and outer thigh muscles to maximize muscle activation. Lower your leg back down to the starting position, returning to the starting position without allowing your knee to touch the ground. Perform the desired number of repetitions on one leg before switching to the other leg. Aim for 10-15 reps per leg, depending on your fitness level. Keep your hips and shoulders stable throughout the exercise, and focus on using the muscles of the outer thigh and glute to lift your leg. The fire hydrant exercise is a simple yet effective way to target the muscles of the outer thigh and glutes, helping to improve hip stability and strengthen the muscles of the lower body. Incorporate it into your lower body workout routine or as a standalone exercise to strengthen and tone your legs.it pairs well with donkey kickbacks, having the same starting position. Adjust the intensity by using resistance bands or ankle weights if desired.

• Banded Clam Shell

The banded clamshell exercise is a great way to target the muscles of the hips, particularly the gluteus medius and gluteus minimus. Begin by lying on your side on a mat or the floor. Bend your knees to approximately 45 degrees and stack them on top of each other. Keep your hips stacked vertically and your head, shoulders, and hips aligned. Place a resistance band just above your knees and pull it taut so that there is resistance when you push against it. Engage your core muscles to help stabilize your torso throughout the exercise and prevent any arching of your lower back. Lift your top knee up towards the ceiling, opening your hips like a clamshell. Keep your feet together and your hips stacked throughout the movement. At the top of the movement, pause for a moment and squeeze your glutes to maximize muscle activation. Avoid rolling your hips back or arching your lower back as you lift your knee. Keep the movement controlled and deliberate to fully engage the muscles. Slowly lower your top knee back down towards the bottom knee, maintaining tension in the resistance band. Perform the desired number of repetitions on one side before switching to the other side. Aim for 10-15 reps per side, depending on your fitness level. The banded clamshell exercise is an effective way to target and strengthen the muscles of the hips, particularly the gluteus medius and gluteus minimus, which are important for hip stability and proper movement mechanics. Incorporate it into your lower body workout routine or as a prehabilitation exercise to help prevent hip and knee injuries. Adjust the resistance of the band as needed to suit your strength level and goals.

- Sumo Squat

The sumo squat is a variation of the traditional squat exercise that targets the muscles of the lower body, including the quadriceps, hamstrings, glutes, and adductors. Begin by standing with your feet wider than shoulder-width apart, toes pointed out at an angle of about 45 degrees. Hold a dumbbell or kettlebell with both hands in front of your body, or place your hands on your hips for balance.Engage your core muscles to help stabilize your torso throughout the exercise and prevent any arching of your lower back. Bend your knees and lower your body down towards the ground, keeping your chest up and your back straight. Imagine sitting back into an imaginary chair. Lower your body down until your thighs are parallel to the ground or as low as is comfortable for you. Keep your knees aligned with your toes and your weight distributed evenly between your heels and the balls of your feet. Push through your heels to return to the starting position, straightening your legs and squeezing your glutes at the top of the movement. At the top of the movement, your legs should be straight but not locked out, and your hips should be fully extended. The sumo squat is an effective exercise for targeting the muscles of the lower body, particularly the inner thighs (adductors), glutes, and quadriceps. It can be incorporated into your lower body workout routine or used as a standalone exercise to strengthen and tone your legs. Adjust the weight used and the depth of the squat to suit your strength level and goals.

- Bulgarian Split Squat

The Bulgarian split squat is a unilateral exercise that primarily targets the muscles of the lower body, including the quadriceps, hamstrings, glutes, and calves. It also engages the core muscles for stability and balance. Begin by placing a bench or elevated surface behind you. Stand facing away from the bench with your feet hip-width apart. Lift one foot and place it behind you on top of the bench, laces down, with the top of your foot resting on the bench. Your other foot should remain planted firmly on the ground in front of you. Engage your core muscles to help stabilize your torso throughout the exercise. Bend your front knee and lower your body towards the ground, keeping your torso upright and your chest up. Your front knee should track over your toes, and your back knee should lower towards the ground. Lower your body down until your front thigh is parallel to the ground or as low as is comfortable for you. Keep your back straight and avoid rounding your shoulders. Push through your front heel to return to the starting position, straightening your front leg and squeezing your glutes at the top of the movement. Perform the desired number of repetitions on one leg before switching to the other leg. Aim for 8-12 reps per leg, depending on your fitness level and goals. Throughout the exercise, focus on maintaining stability in your core and avoiding any excessive movement or shifting of your hips. Keep your shoulders square and your spine in a neutral position. The Bulgarian split squat is an effective exercise for building strength and muscle mass in the lower body, as well as improving balance and stability. It can be incorporated into your leg workout routine or used as a unilateral exercise to address muscle imbalances between the left and right sides of the body. Adjust the height of the bench or surface to increase or decrease the difficulty of the exercise, and consider holding dumbbells or kettlebells for added resistance.

- Hip Thrust

The hip thrust is a highly effective exercise for targeting and strengthening the muscles of the glutes, hamstrings, and lower back. Begin by sitting on the ground with your upper back against a sturdy bench or elevated surface. Your knees should be bent, and your feet flat on the floor about hip-width apart. You can optionally place dumbbells or a padded barbell across your hips for added resistance. Roll the barbell over your hips, or place a weight plate or resistance band just above your hips. This will be the resistance you'll lift during the exercise. Ensure that your shoulder blades are resting firmly against the bench. Engage your core muscles to help stabilize your torso throughout the exercise. Press through your heels and lift your hips towards the ceiling, squeezing your glutes at the top of the movement. Focus on pushing your hips as high as possible without overarching your lower back. At the top of the movement, your body should form a straight line from your shoulders to your knees. Pause for a moment to squeeze your glutes and maximize muscle activation. Slowly lower your hips back down towards the ground, maintaining tension in your glutes and hamstrings throughout the movement. The hip thrust is an excellent exercise for targeting and strengthening the glutes, hamstrings, and lower back muscles. It can be incorporated into your lower body workout routine as a primary exercise or used as a supplementary exercise to enhance glute activation and development. Adjust the weight of the barbell, dumbbells or resistance band to suit your strength level and ensure proper form throughout the exercise.

7

Leg Exercises

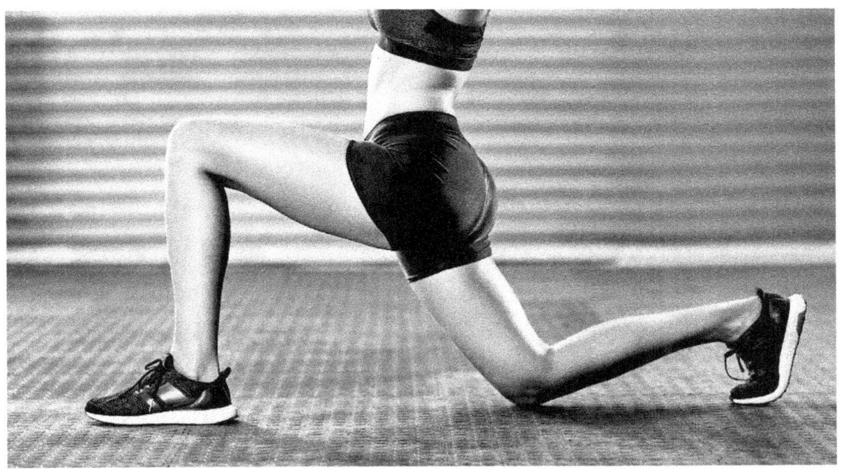

- Body weight Squat

The squat is a fundamental compound exercise that targets multiple muscles in the lower body, including the quadriceps, hamstrings, glutes, and calves, while also engaging the core and lower back muscles for stability. Stand tall with your feet shoulder-width apart or slightly wider. Your toes can be pointed slightly outward to accommodate your natural hip and ankle mobility. Keep your chest up, shoulders back, and core engaged throughout the movement. Bend your knees and lower your body down towards the ground, as if you're sitting back into an imaginary chair. Keep your weight on your heels and your knees tracking in line with your toes. Aim to lower your hips until your thighs are parallel to the ground, or as low as your mobility allows while maintaining proper form. The depth of your squat will depend on your flexibility and mobility. Focus on achieving a depth where your thighs are parallel to the ground while keeping your heels flat on the floor and your chest up. Avoid letting your knees collapse inward or leaning too far forward with your torso. Push through your heels to return to the starting position, straightening your legs and squeezing your glutes at the top of the movement. Focus on driving your hips forward to engage the glutes and maintain a neutral spine. At the top of the movement, your hips should be fully extended, and your body should be in a straight line from your head to your heels. Avoid hyperextending your lower back or locking out your knees. Perform the desired number of repetitions, aiming for 8-12 reps, depending on your fitness level and goals. The squat is a versatile exercise that can be performed with just your body weight or with added resistance such as dumbbells, barbells, or kettlebells to increase the challenge. It's important to start with proper form and gradually increase the intensity and load as you become stronger and more proficient with the movement. Squats are a fundamental movement pattern that can be incorporated into any lower body workout routine to build strength, muscle mass, and functional movement capacity.

- Lunges

The lunge is a versatile lower body exercise that targets multiple muscle groups, including the quadriceps, hamstrings, glutes, and calves. It also engages the core muscles for stability and balance. Stand tall with your feet together and your arms at your sides. Take a big step forward with your right foot, landing with your heel first and then rolling onto the ball of your foot. Keep your torso upright, your chest up, and your shoulders back throughout the movement. Bend both knees to lower your body towards the ground, aiming to bring your front thigh parallel to the floor. Your front knee should be directly above your ankle, and your back knee should hover just above the ground. The depth of your lunge will depend on your flexibility and mobility. Aim to lower your body until your front thigh is parallel to the ground, or as low as is comfortable for you, while maintaining proper form. Push through the heel of your front foot to return to the starting position, straightening your front leg and bringing your back foot forward to meet your front foot. Perform the same movement with your left leg, stepping forward into a lunge and then returning to the starting position. Continue alternating legs for the desired number of repetitions, aiming for 8-12 reps per leg, depending on your fitness level and goals. The lunge can be performed with just your body weight or with added resistance such as dumbbells, barbells, or kettlebells to increase the challenge. It's important to start with proper form and gradually increase the intensity and load as you become stronger and more proficient with the movement. Lunges are a functional exercise that can be incorporated into any lower body workout routine to improve strength, stability, and balance.

- Reverse Lunge

The reverse lunge is a variation of the traditional lunge exercise that targets similar muscle groups but places slightly different emphasis on the lower body and core. Stand tall with your feet together and your arms at your sides. Take a big step backward with your right foot, landing with the ball of your foot first and then lowering your heel towards the ground. Keep your torso upright, your chest up, and your shoulders back throughout the movement. Bend both knees to lower your body towards the ground, aiming to bring your back knee just above the ground. Your front knee should be directly above your ankle, and your back knee should hover just above the ground. The depth of your lunge will depend on your flexibility and mobility. Aim to lower your body until your back knee is just above the ground, or as low as is comfortable for you, while maintaining proper form. Push through the heel of your front foot to return to the starting position, straightening your front leg and bringing your back foot forward to meet your front foot. Perform the same movement with your left leg, stepping backward into a lunge and then returning to the starting position. Continue alternating legs for the desired number of repetitions, aiming for 8-12 reps per leg, depending on your fitness level and goals. The reverse lunge can be performed with just your body weight or with added resistance such as dumbbells, barbells, or kettlebells to increase the challenge. It's important to start with proper form and gradually increase the intensity and load as you become stronger and more proficient with the movement. Reverse lunges are a functional exercise that can help improve strength, stability, and balance in the lower body and core.

- One-leg Squat

The one-leg squat, also known as the pistol squat, is an advanced body weight exercise that targets the muscles of the lower body, including the quadriceps, hamstrings, glutes, and calves, as well as the core for stability and balance. Stand tall with your feet together and your arms at your sides. Shift your weight onto one leg and extend your other leg out in front of you. Keep your foot flexed and your toes pointed upward throughout the movement. Engage your core muscles to help stabilize your torso throughout the exercise. Bend your standing leg and lower your body towards the ground, keeping your chest up and your back straight. Imagine sitting back into an imaginary chair. Lower your body down as far as you can while maintaining balance and control. Aim to lower your hips until your thigh is parallel to the ground, or as low as is comfortable for you, while keeping your heel flat on the ground. Push through your heel to return to the starting position, straightening your leg and squeezing your glutes at the top of the movement. Perform the same movement on the opposite leg, shifting your weight onto the other leg and extending the other leg out in front of you. Continue alternating legs for the desired number of repetitions, aiming for 5-10 reps per leg, depending on your fitness level and goals. The one-leg squat requires significant strength, balance, and flexibility, so it's important to start with proper form and gradually increase the difficulty as you become stronger and more proficient with the movement. You can use a chair or bench for assistance or hold onto a support for balance if needed. As you progress, you can increase the challenge by performing the exercise on an elevated surface or holding onto weights for added resistance.

- Wall sit

The wall sit is an isometric exercise that primarily targets the quadriceps, but also engages the glutes, hamstrings, and calves. It's a simple yet effective exercise that can be done virtually anywhere with just a wall. Find a clear wall space and stand with your back against the wall. Walk your feet out slightly in front of you, about shoulder-width apart. Your feet should be positioned approximately 1-2 feet away from the wall. Slowly slide your back down the wall, bending your knees until they are at a 90-degree angle. Your thighs should be parallel to the ground, and your knees should be directly above your ankles. Press your lower back firmly against the wall and ensure that your entire back is supported. Engage your core muscles to help stabilize your torso throughout the exercise. Hold this position for as long as you can, aiming for 20-60 seconds initially. As you become stronger, you can gradually increase the duration of the hold. Ensure that your knees are aligned with your ankles and not protruding over your toes. Keep your chest up and your shoulders back, and avoid leaning forward or rounding your back. When you're ready to finish, slowly push yourself back up the wall by straightening your legs. Rest for a moment before repeating the exercise for additional sets or duration. The wall sit is an effective way to build lower body strength, endurance, and stability. It's particularly beneficial for athletes involved in sports that require lower body strength and endurance, such as skiing, basketball, and cycling. You can make the wall sit more challenging by holding weights on your thighs or increasing the duration of the hold over time.

- Side Lunge

The side lunge is a dynamic lower body exercise that primarily targets the muscles of the inner and outer thighs (adductors and abductors), glutes, hamstrings, and quadriceps. Begin by standing tall with your feet together and your arms at your sides. Take a large step to the right with your right foot, keeping your toes pointed forward and your left foot stationary. Shift your body weight to your right leg as you bend your right knee and lower your body down towards the ground. Your right knee should track in line with your toes, and your left leg should remain straight. Keep your chest up and your back straight throughout the movement. Lower your body down as far as is comfortable for you, aiming to bring your right thigh parallel to the ground. Keep your right knee aligned with your ankle and avoid letting it collapse inward. Push through your right heel to return to the starting position, straightening your right leg and bringing your left foot back to meet your right foot. Perform the same movement on the opposite side, taking a large step to the left with your left foot and lowering your body down into a lunge. Continue alternating sides for the desired number of repetitions, aiming for 8-12 reps per leg, depending on your fitness level and goals. The side lunge is a great exercise for targeting the muscles of the inner and outer thighs, as well as the glutes and hamstrings. It's a functional movement that can help improve lateral strength, stability, and mobility, making it beneficial for sports and activities that involve side-to-side movements. You can perform side lunges with just your body weight or add resistance by holding dumbbells or a kettlebell for added challenge.

- Calf Raises

Calf raises are a simple yet effective exercise for targeting the muscles of the calves, specifically the gastrocnemius and soleus muscles. Stand tall with your feet hip-width apart and your arms at your sides or holding onto a stable surface for balance, such as a wall or a chair. Engage your core muscles to help stabilize your torso throughout the exercise. Slowly rise up onto the balls of your feet by lifting your heels off the ground as high as you can. Focus on using your calf muscles to lift your body weight. At the top of the movement, pause for a moment and squeeze your calf muscles to maximize muscle activation. Lower your heels back down towards the ground in a controlled manner, until your heels are just below the level of your toes. Aim to lower your heels until you feel a stretch in your calf muscles, then push back up to the starting position. Avoid bouncing at the bottom of the movement. Perform the desired number of repetitions, aiming for 12-15 reps, depending on your fitness level and goals. Calf raises can be performed using just your body weight, or you can add resistance by holding dumbbells or using a calf raise machine at the gym. You can also vary the exercise by performing single-leg calf raises or standing on a step or raised platform to increase the range of motion. Including calf raises in your workout routine can help improve calf strength, muscle tone, and ankle stability, which are important for various daily activities and athletic pursuits.

- Kettlebell Swing

The kettlebell swing is a dynamic and powerful exercise that targets multiple muscle groups, including the glutes, hamstrings, lower back, shoulders, and core. It's a functional movement that mimics activities like lifting, jumping, and sprinting, making it a valuable addition to any strength training or conditioning program. Stand with your feet slightly wider than shoulder-width apart, toes pointed slightly outward. Place a kettlebell on the floor about a foot in front of you. Bend at the hips and grasp the kettlebell handle with both hands, keeping your back flat and your chest up. Your arms should be straight, and your shoulders should be pulled back and down. Initiate the movement by driving your hips back and swinging the kettlebell between your legs, similar to a hike pass in football. Keep your arms relaxed and allow the kettlebell to swing freely. Explosively drive your hips forward and stand up tall, swinging the kettlebell up to shoulder height or slightly above. Your arms should remain straight throughout the movement, with the momentum generated by your hips. At the top of the movement, your body should form a straight line from your head to your heels, with your glutes fully engaged. Squeeze your glutes and contract your core muscles to maintain stability. Allow the kettlebell to swing back down between your legs as you hinge at the hips again, keeping your back flat and your chest up. Your arms should act as a pendulum, with the power generated from your hips. Perform the kettlebell swing for the desired number of repetitions, aiming for 10-15 reps per set, depending on your fitness level and goals. It's essential to use proper form and technique when performing the kettlebell swing to prevent injury and maximize effectiveness. Start with a light kettlebell to practice the movement and gradually increase the weight as you become more comfortable and proficient. Avoid using your arms to lift the kettlebell and focus on generating power from your hips. The kettlebell swing is a versatile exercise that can be incorporated into full-body workouts, circuit training, or conditioning routines to improve strength, power, and cardiovascular fitness.

- Goblet Squat

The goblet squat is a highly effective lower body exercise that targets the quadriceps, hamstrings, glutes, and core muscles. It's performed with a dumbbell or kettlebell held at chest level, which helps to counterbalance the movement and keep the torso upright. Stand with your feet slightly wider than shoulder-width apart and your toes pointed slightly outward. Hold a dumbbell or kettlebell vertically with both hands, close to your chest. Your elbows should be bent and pointing down. Engage your core muscles to help stabilize your torso throughout the exercise. Bend your knees and lower your body down into a squat position, keeping your chest up and your back straight. Imagine sitting back into an imaginary chair. Lower your body down until your thighs are parallel to the ground, or as low as is comfortable for you while maintaining proper form. Keep your knees aligned with your toes and your weight on your heels. Push through your heels to return to the starting position, straightening your legs and squeezing your glutes at the top of the movement. At the top of the movement, your legs should be straight but not locked out, and your hips should be fully extended. Perform the desired number of repetitions, aiming for 8-12 reps, depending on your fitness level and goals. The goblet squat is a great exercise for building lower body strength, improving squat mechanics, and enhancing core stability. Holding the weight at chest level helps to promote an upright torso position and encourages proper alignment throughout the movement. It's suitable for individuals of all fitness levels and can be easily modified by adjusting the weight used. Incorporate goblet squats into your lower body workout routine to develop functional strength and muscle tone in the legs, glutes, and core.

8

Conclusion

There are many exercises you can do at home with just your body weight. Whe you add dumbbells and resistance bands the options are opened up even more. Any exercise done without added weight can always be modified to add weight and more of a challenge. You really can get a good full body, all around exercise from home, you just need to know how. All of the exercises in this book can be put together in a variety of ways to make a unique workout routine. It's important to warm up and to cool down before and after exercising. Always remember to exercise both sides or your body when doing a movement that isolates one side of your body.

If you enjoyed this book or found it useful, leave me a 5-Star review on Amazon and let me know what you liked! It helps me out a lot and doesn't take long to do.